The LifeChanger 90-Day Food Journal

For The Ketogenic Diet And Intermittent Fasting

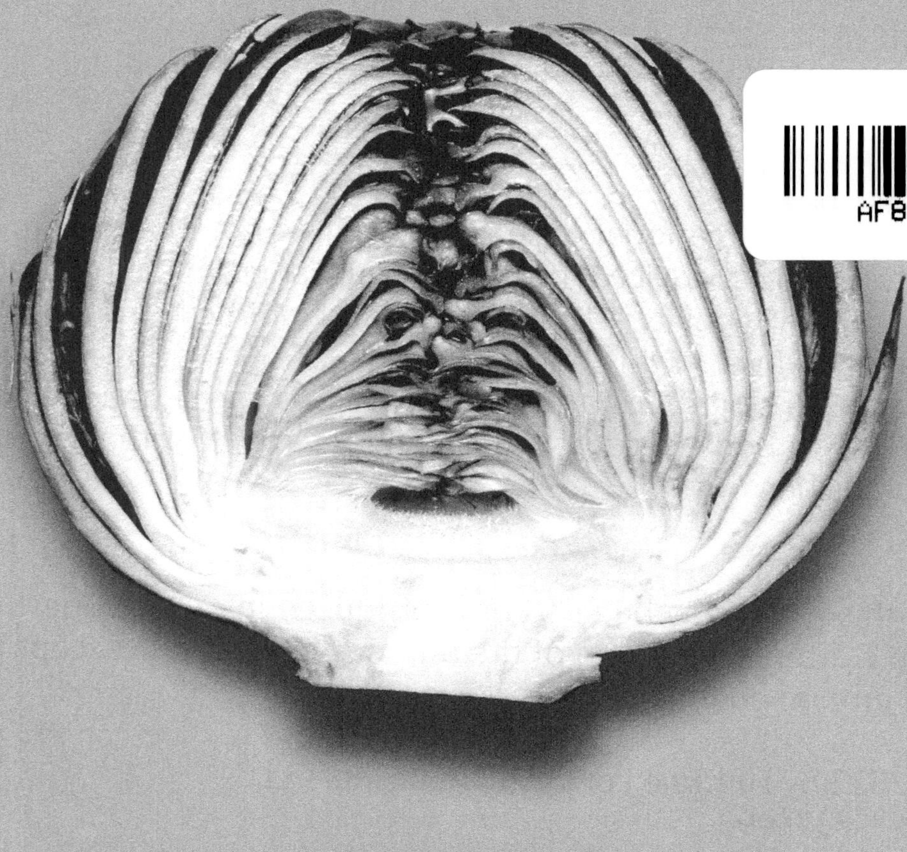

Nancy Ducharme
Sharon Merriman, RWP

This book is for informational purposes only. It is not intended to serve as a substitute for medical advice. The author, publisher, and all affiliated parties disclaim any and all liability arising directly and indirectly from the use of any information contained in this book. A health care practitioner should always be consulted regarding speciÞc medical conditions and situations. Any product mentioned in this book does not imply endorsement of that product by the author or publisher.

ISBN#; 978-1-7371093-2-7

Introduction

This 90-day food journal is meant for those who are following the ketogenic diet as a tool to help control, or reverse, certain metabolic conditions such as pre-diabetes, type 2 diabetes, cancer, and obesity. This easy-to-use daily tracker will help you stay on top of your macros (total calories, carbohydrates, and protein) and the start/stop times for fasting windows. You can also track water intake and your Glucose-Ketone Index number (more on this later) for those who are using this diet to control cancer.

In addition to the keto diet, intermittent fasting can be added to enhance results. Fasting is not about starving yourself. It's a therapeutic method used since ancient times to support wellness. When done correctly, it can boost the immune system and raise the level of ketone bodies in the blood by "flipping the switch" from burning sugar to burning fat for fuel. Fasting also promotes autophagy which is the body's way of cleaning out damaged cells to regenerate new, healthy cells.

Incorporating this approach has helped thousands of people take control of their wellness and reverse obesity and type 2 diabetes through the regulation of blood sugar and catabolic hormones. Intermittent fasting will help do the same for patients with cancer. Many books have been released explaining the benefits of intermittent fasting including two of my personal favorites, Dr. Jason Fung's best-sellers, "*The Obesity Code" and his "Complete Guide to Fasting*".

While a ketogenic diet combined with intermittent fasting can be a valuable tool to reverse many diseases, it is important to note that there are certain people who should not participate in this regimen. Cancer patients who have the B-RAF V600E gene mutation should not be on a ketogenic diet because it could act as a catalyst for cancer growth. Following this diet, also poses a risk to people who have type 1 diabetes. Therefore, you should always consult your physician before starting any type of therapeutic diet.

The Glucose-Ketone Index

(This is specifically meant for people who are in the process of reversing cancer, pre-diabetes, or type 2 diabetes.)

The Glucose-Ketone Index (GKI) is a measurement devised by Thomas Seyfried Ph.D., a cancer researcher and biology professor at Boston College. This is an excellent tool used to monitor the amount of ketone bodies in the bloodstream. There is an entire chapter written about this in my book, "*Lifechanger: How to Starve Cancer Using Metabolic Strategies and Deep Therapeutic Ketosis*".

For cancer patients, ketone bodies are important because they are HDAC inhibitors. HDAC is an acronym for histone deacetylase inhibitors - a new class of anti-cancer agents that interrupt the development of cancer. Pharmaceutical companies are in the process of developing drugs which mimic HDAC inhibitors, but we can naturally produce our own by optimizing ketone body production through a therapeutic ketogenic diet.

To record your GKI requires testing your fasting blood-sugar as well as your ketone level. This can be done in one easy step by using a blood monitor called the Keto Mojo monitor which is available through my site nancyducharme.com.

Once you get both numbers you divide your glucose number by 18. Cut it off at the hundredth's decimal for accuracy. Next, take that new number and divide it by your keto score and you will have your Glucose-Ketone Index number. Your goal is to be at 3 or lower to get into the optimal zone for ketosis.

In the upper right corner of the journal page, you will see a space for your GKI number for morning, midday, and evening.

Filling Out Your Daily Journal

Begin by filling in the date and the day. Enter the time when you broke your fast. You can then log in what you broke your fast with. There is plenty of space to write down your details. Next, fill in the macros for that meal.

As the day progresses you can log in other meals and beverages you've consumed during your eating window. There is also a space to keep track of water consumption. Finally, log in the exact time you resumed your fasting.

Flip the page and you will see ample space for journaling. What went right for you, what didn't, and how you can make changes – feel free to write about your emotional journey as well.

Remember, what you put into your head matters…

~ ***Nancy***

FASTING & FOOD LOG

Glucose-Ketone Index #

AM ....

MID-DAY ....

PM ....

Date: ______________

[I Broke My Fast At: ________ a.m. p.m.]

M T W T F S S

["Every step is a step toward being better." Sharon Merriman]

(I Broke My Fast With...)

ITEM	CALORIES	FAT	NET CARBS	PROTEIN

(Other Meals Eaten Today)

ITEM	CALORIES	FAT	NET CARBS	PROTEIN

Water Intake

[I Resumed Fasting At This Time]

What Went Well For Me Today

What Didn't Go Well For Me Today

How I Can Make It Better

FASTING & FOOD LOG

Date: ______________

[I Broke My Fast At: ________ a.m. p.m.]

M T W T F S S

Glucose-Ketone Index #

AM ....

MID-DAY ....

PM ....

["Be the change that you wish to see in the world." Mahatma Gandhi]

(I Broke My Fast With...)

ITEM	CALORIES	FAT	NET CARBS	PROTEIN

(Other Meals Eaten Today)

ITEM	CALORIES	FAT	NET CARBS	PROTEIN

Water Intake

[I Resumed Fasting At This Time]

What Went Well For Me Today

What Didn't Go Well For Me Today

How I Can Make It Better

FASTING & FOOD LOG

Date: ____________________

M T W T F S S

[I Broke My Fast At: __________ a.m. p.m.]

Glucose-Ketone Index #

AM ....

MID-DAY ....

PM ....

["I have not failed. I've just found 10,000 ways that don't work." Thomas A. Edison]

(I Broke My Fast With...)

ITEM	CALORIES	FAT	NET CARBS	PROTEIN

(Other Meals Eaten Today)

ITEM	CALORIES	FAT	NET CARBS	PROTEIN

[I Resumed Fasting At This Time]

Water Intake

What Went Well For Me Today

What Didn't Go Well For Me Today

How I Can Make It Better

FASTING & FOOD LOG

Glucose-Ketone Index #

AM ....

MID-DAY ....

PM ....

Date: ______________

[I Broke My Fast At: ________ a.m. p.m.]

M T W T F S S

["It is never too later to be what you might have been." George Eliot]

(I Broke My Fast With...)

ITEM	CALORIES	FAT	NET CARBS	PROTEIN

(Other Meals Eaten Today)

ITEM	CALORIES	FAT	NET CARBS	PROTEIN

[I Resumed Fasting At This Time]

Water Intake

What Went Well For Me Today

What Didn't Go Well For Me Today

How I Can Make It Better

FASTING & FOOD LOG

Glucose-Ketone Index #

AM ....

MID-DAY ....

PM ....

Date: ______________

[I Broke My Fast At: ________ a.m. p.m.]

M T W T F S S

["Life isn't about finding yourself. Life is about creating yourself." George Bernard Shaw]

(I Broke My Fast With...)

ITEM	CALORIES	FAT	NET CARBS	PROTEIN

(Other Meals Eaten Today)

ITEM	CALORIES	FAT	NET CARBS	PROTEIN

[I Resumed Fasting At This Time]

Water Intake

What Went Well For Me Today

What Didn't Go Well For Me Today

How I Can Make It Better

FASTING & FOOD LOG

Glucose-Ketone Index #

AM ....

MID-DAY ....

PM ....

Date: ______________

[I Broke My Fast At: ________ a.m. p.m.]

M T W T F S S

["Success is not final, failure is not fatal: it is the courage to continue that courts."
Winston S. Churchill]

I Broke My Fast With...

ITEM	CALORIES	FAT	NET CARBS	PROTEIN

Other Meals Eaten Today

ITEM	CALORIES	FAT	NET CARBS	PROTEIN

Water Intake

I Resumed Fasting At This Time

What Went Well For Me Today

What Didn't Go Well For Me Today

How I Can Make It Better

FASTING & FOOD LOG

Glucose-Ketone Index #

AM ....

MID-DAY ....

PM ....

Date: ____________

[I Broke My Fast At: ________ a.m. p.m.]

M T W T F S S

["What drains your spirit drains your body. What fuels your spirit fuels your body."]
Caroline Myss

(I Broke My Fast With...)

ITEM	CALORIES	FAT	NET CARBS	PROTEIN

(Other Meals Eaten Today)

ITEM	CALORIES	FAT	NET CARBS	PROTEIN

Water Intake

[I Resumed Fasting At This Time]

What Went Well For Me Today

What Didn't Go Well For Me Today

How I Can Make It Better

FASTING & FOOD LOG

Date: ______________ [I Broke My Fast At: __________ a.m. p.m.]

Glucose-Ketone Index #

AM ....

MID-DAY ....

PM ....

M T W T F S S

["It is health that is real wealth and not pieces of gold and silver." Mahatma Gandhi]

(I Broke My Fast With...)

ITEM	CALORIES	FAT	NET CARBS	PROTEIN

(Other Meals Eaten Today)

ITEM	CALORIES	FAT	NET CARBS	PROTEIN

Water Intake

[I Resumed Fasting At This Time]

What Went Well For Me Today

What Didn't Go Well For Me Today

How I Can Make It Better

FASTING & FOOD LOG

Date: ______________ [I Broke My Fast At: __________ a.m. p.m.]

M T W T F S S

Glucose-Ketone Index #

AM ....

MID-DAY ....

PM ....

["He who has health has hope and he who has hope has everything." Arabian Proverb]

I Broke My Fast With...

ITEM	CALORIES	FAT	NET CARBS	PROTEIN

Other Meals Eaten Today

ITEM	CALORIES	FAT	NET CARBS	PROTEIN

Water Intake

[I Resumed Fasting At This Time]

What Went Well For Me Today

What Didn't Go Well For Me Today

How I Can Make It Better

FASTING & FOOD LOG

Glucose-Ketone Index #

AM ....

MID-DAY ....

PM ....

Date: ______________

[I Broke My Fast At: ________ a.m. p.m.]

M T W T F S S

["A healthy outside starts from the inside." Robert Urich]

I Broke My Fast With...

ITEM	CALORIES	FAT	NET CARBS	PROTEIN

Other Meals Eaten Today

ITEM	CALORIES	FAT	NET CARBS	PROTEIN

Water Intake

[I Resumed Fasting At This Time]

What Went Well For Me Today

What Didn't Go Well For Me Today

How I Can Make It Better

FASTING & FOOD LOG

Date: ________________ [I Broke My Fast At: ________ a.m. p.m.]

M T W T F S S

Glucose-Ketone Index #	
AM	....
MID-DAY	....
PM	....

["Wellness is a connection of paths: Knowledge and Action." Joshua Holtz]

(I Broke My Fast With...)

ITEM	CALORIES	FAT	NET CARBS	PROTEIN

(Other Meals Eaten Today)

ITEM	CALORIES	FAT	NET CARBS	PROTEIN

Water Intake

[I Resumed Fasting At This Time]

What Went Well For Me Today

What Didn't Go Well For Me Today

How I Can Make It Better

FASTING & FOOD LOG

Glucose-Ketone Index #

AM ....

MID-DAY ....

PM ....

Date: ________________

[I Broke My Fast At: __________ a.m. p.m.]

M T W T F S S

["It's no coincidence that four of the six letters in health heal." Ed Northstrum]

I Broke My Fast With...

ITEM	CALORIES	FAT	NET CARBS	PROTEIN

Other Meals Eaten Today

ITEM	CALORIES	FAT	NET CARBS	PROTEIN

Water Intake

I Resumed Fasting At This Time

What Went Well For Me Today

What Didn't Go Well For Me Today

How I Can Make It Better

FASTING & FOOD LOG

Date: ________________

[I Broke My Fast At: __________ a.m. p.m.]

M T W T F S S

Glucose-Ketone Index #

AM ....

MID-DAY ....

PM ....

["The key to a healthy life is having a healthy mind." Richard Davidson]

(I Broke My Fast With...)

ITEM	CALORIES	FAT	NET CARBS	PROTEIN

(Other Meals Eaten Today)

ITEM	CALORIES	FAT	NET CARBS	PROTEIN

Water Intake

[I Resumed Fasting At This Time]

What Went Well For Me Today

What Didn't Go Well For Me Today

How I Can Make It Better

FASTING & FOOD LOG

Glucose-Ketone Index #

AM ....

MID-DAY ....

PM ....

Date: ________________

[I Broke My Fast At: ________ a.m. p.m.]

M T W T F S S

["The groundwork for all happiness is good health." Leigh Hunt]

(I Broke My Fast With...)

ITEM	CALORIES	FAT	NET CARBS	PROTEIN

(Other Meals Eaten Today)

ITEM	CALORIES	FAT	NET CARBS	PROTEIN

[I Resumed Fasting At This Time]

Water Intake

What Went Well For Me Today

What Didn't Go Well For Me Today

How I Can Make It Better

FASTING & FOOD LOG

Date: ____________ [I Broke My Fast At: ________ a.m. p.m.]

M T W T F S S

Glucose-Ketone Index #

AM ....

MID-DAY ....

PM ....

["Laughing decreases blood pressure and increases blood flow." Unknown]

I Broke My Fast With...

ITEM	CALORIES	FAT	NET CARBS	PROTEIN

Other Meals Eaten Today

ITEM	CALORIES	FAT	NET CARBS	PROTEIN

[I Resumed Fasting At This Time]

Water Intake

What Went Well For Me Today

What Didn't Go Well For Me Today

How I Can Make It Better

FASTING & FOOD LOG

Date: ______________

M T W T F S S

[I Broke My Fast At: __________ a.m. p.m.]

Glucose-Ketone Index #

AM ....

MID-DAY ....

PM ....

["Health is worth more than learning." Thomas Jefferson]

(I Broke My Fast With...)

ITEM	CALORIES	FAT	NET CARBS	PROTEIN

(Other Meals Eaten Today)

ITEM	CALORIES	FAT	NET CARBS	PROTEIN

Water Intake

[I Resumed Fasting At This Time]

What Went Well For Me Today

What Didn't Go Well For Me Today

How I Can Make It Better

FASTING & FOOD LOG

Date: ______________

[I Broke My Fast At: ________ a.m. p.m.]

M T W T F S S

Glucose-Ketone Index #	
AM	....
MID-DAY	....
PM	....

["Your body hears everything your mind says." Naomi Judd]

(I Broke My Fast With...)

ITEM	CALORIES	FAT	NET CARBS	PROTEIN

(Other Meals Eaten Today)

ITEM	CALORIES	FAT	NET CARBS	PROTEIN

Water Intake

[I Resumed Fasting At This Time]

What Went Well For Me Today

What Didn't Go Well For Me Today

How I Can Make It Better

FASTING & FOOD LOG

Date: ______________

[I Broke My Fast At: ________ a.m. p.m.]

M T W T F S S

Glucose-Ketone Index #

AM ....

MID-DAY ....

PM ....

["Your illness is not your identity. Your chemistry is not your character." Pastor Rick Warren]

(I Broke My Fast With...)

ITEM	CALORIES	FAT	NET CARBS	PROTEIN

(Other Meals Eaten Today)

ITEM	CALORIES	FAT	NET CARBS	PROTEIN

Water Intake

[I Resumed Fasting At This Time]

What Went Well For Me Today

What Didn't Go Well For Me Today

How I Can Make It Better

FASTING & FOOD LOG

Date: ____________ [I Broke My Fast At: ________ a.m. p.m.]

M T W T F S S

Glucose-Ketone Index #

AM ....
MID-DAY ....
PM ....

["You can't stop the waves, but you can learn to surf." Jon Kabat-Zinn]

(I Broke My Fast With...)

ITEM	CALORIES	FAT	NET CARBS	PROTEIN

(Other Meals Eaten Today)

ITEM	CALORIES	FAT	NET CARBS	PROTEIN

Water Intake

[I Resumed Fasting At This Time]

What Went Well For Me Today

What Didn't Go Well For Me Today

How I Can Make It Better

FASTING & FOOD LOG

Glucose-Ketone Index #

AM ....

MID-DAY ....

PM ....

Date: ____________

[I Broke My Fast At: ________ a.m. p.m.]

M T W T F S S

["The stream of life is a wave on the ocean of love." Maharishi Mahesh Yogi]

(I Broke My Fast With...)

ITEM	CALORIES	FAT	NET CARBS	PROTEIN

(Other Meals Eaten Today)

ITEM	CALORIES	FAT	NET CARBS	PROTEIN

[I Resumed Fasting At This Time]

Water Intake

What Went Well For Me Today

What Didn't Go Well For Me Today

How I Can Make It Better

FASTING & FOOD LOG

Glucose-Ketone Index #

AM ....

MID-DAY ....

PM ....

Date: ______________ [I Broke My Fast At: ________ a.m. p.m.]

M T W T F S S

["Set your life on fire, seek those who fan your flames." Rumi]

(I Broke My Fast With...)

ITEM	CALORIES	FAT	NET CARBS	PROTEIN

(Other Meals Eaten Today)

ITEM	CALORIES	FAT	NET CARBS	PROTEIN

[I Resumed Fasting At This Time]

Water Intake

What Went Well For Me Today

What Didn't Go Well For Me Today

How I Can Make It Better

FASTING & FOOD LOG

Date: ______________ [I Broke My Fast At: __________ a.m. p.m.]

M T W T F S S

Glucose-Ketone Index #

AM ....

MID-DAY ....

PM ....

["Of all fires, love is the only inexhaustible one." Pablo Neruda]

(I Broke My Fast With...)

ITEM	CALORIES	FAT	NET CARBS	PROTEIN

(Other Meals Eaten Today)

ITEM	CALORIES	FAT	NET CARBS	PROTEIN

Water Intake

[I Resumed Fasting At This Time]

What Went Well For Me Today

What Didn't Go Well For Me Today

How I Can Make It Better

FASTING & FOOD LOG

Date: ______________

[I Broke My Fast At: ________ a.m. p.m.]

M T W T F S S

Glucose-Ketone Index #

AM ....

MID-DAY ....

PM ....

["The mind is not a vessel to be filled, but a fore to be kindled." Plutarch]

(I Broke My Fast With...)

ITEM	CALORIES	FAT	NET CARBS	PROTEIN

(Other Meals Eaten Today)

ITEM	CALORIES	FAT	NET CARBS	PROTEIN

Water Intake

[I Resumed Fasting At This Time]

What Went Well For Me Today

What Didn't Go Well For Me Today

How I Can Make It Better

FASTING & FOOD LOG

Date: ____________________

[I Broke My Fast At: __________ a.m. p.m.]

M T W T F S S

Glucose-Ketone Index #

AM ....

MID-DAY ....

PM ....

["Look deep into nature, and then you will understand everything better." Albert Einstein]

(I Broke My Fast With...)

ITEM	CALORIES	FAT	NET CARBS	PROTEIN

(Other Meals Eaten Today)

ITEM	CALORIES	FAT	NET CARBS	PROTEIN

Water Intake

[I Resumed Fasting At This Time]

What Went Well For Me Today

What Didn't Go Well For Me Today

How I Can Make It Better

FASTING & FOOD LOG

Date: ____________ [I Broke My Fast At: ________ a.m. p.m.]

M T W T F S S

Glucose-Ketone Index #

AM ....

MID-DAY ....

PM ....

["Nature does not hurry, yet everything is accomplished." Lao Tzu]

(I Broke My Fast With...)

ITEM	CALORIES	FAT	NET CARBS	PROTEIN

(Other Meals Eaten Today)

ITEM	CALORIES	FAT	NET CARBS	PROTEIN

[I Resumed Fasting At This Time]

Water Intake

What Went Well For Me Today

What Didn't Go Well For Me Today

How I Can Make It Better

FASTING & FOOD LOG

Date: ________________

I Broke My Fast At: __________ a.m. p.m.

M T W T F S S

Glucose-Ketone Index #

AM ....

MID-DAY ....

PM ....

"If you truly love nature, you will find beauty everywhere." Laura Ingalls Wilder

I Broke My Fast With...

ITEM	CALORIES	FAT	NET CARBS	PROTEIN

Other Meals Eaten Today

ITEM	CALORIES	FAT	NET CARBS	PROTEIN

Water Intake

I Resumed Fasting At This Time

What Went Well For Me Today

What Didn't Go Well For Me Today

How I Can Make It Better

FASTING & FOOD LOG

Date: ______________ [I Broke My Fast At: ________ a.m. p.m.]

M T W T F S S

Glucose-Ketone Index #

AM ....

MID-DAY ....

PM ....

["I go to nature to be soothed and healed, and to have my sense put in order."]
John Burroughs

(I Broke My Fast With...)

ITEM	CALORIES	FAT	NET CARBS	PROTEIN

(Other Meals Eaten Today)

ITEM	CALORIES	FAT	NET CARBS	PROTEIN

Water Intake

[I Resumed Fasting At This Time]

What Went Well For Me Today

What Didn't Go Well For Me Today

How I Can Make It Better

FASTING & FOOD LOG

Date: ________________ [I Broke My Fast At: __________ a.m. p.m.]

M T W T F S S

Glucose-Ketone Index #

AM ....

MID-DAY ....

PM ....

["Everything in nature invites us constantly to be what we are." Great Ehrlich]

(I Broke My Fast With...)

ITEM	CALORIES	FAT	NET CARBS	PROTEIN

(Other Meals Eaten Today)

ITEM	CALORIES	FAT	NET CARBS	PROTEIN

Water Intake

[I Resumed Fasting At This Time]

What Went Well For Me Today

What Didn't Go Well For Me Today

How I Can Make It Better

FASTING & FOOD LOG

Date: ______________ [I Broke My Fast At: ________ a.m. p.m.]

M T W T F S S

Glucose-Ketone Index #

AM ....

MID-DAY ....

PM ....

["Spring is nature's way of saying, 'Let's party!'" Robin Williams]

(I Broke My Fast With...)

ITEM	CALORIES	FAT	NET CARBS	PROTEIN

(Other Meals Eaten Today)

ITEM	CALORIES	FAT	NET CARBS	PROTEIN

Water Intake

[I Resumed Fasting At This Time]

What Went Well For Me Today

What Didn't Go Well For Me Today

How I Can Make It Better

FASTING & FOOD LOG

Date: ______________

M T W T F S S

[I Broke My Fast At: ________ a.m. p.m.]

Glucose-Ketone Index #

AM ....

MID-DAY ....

PM ....

["The earth has music for those who listen." William Shakespeare]

I Broke My Fast With...

ITEM	CALORIES	FAT	NET CARBS	PROTEIN

Other Meals Eaten Today

ITEM	CALORIES	FAT	NET CARBS	PROTEIN

Water Intake

[I Resumed Fasting At This Time]

What Went Well For Me Today

What Didn't Go Well For Me Today

How I Can Make It Better

FASTING & FOOD LOG

Date: ____________

[I Broke My Fast At: ________ a.m. p.m.]

M T W T F S S

Glucose-Ketone Index #

AM ....

MID-DAY ....

PM ....

["A weed is not more than a flower in disguise." James Russell Lowell]

(I Broke My Fast With...)

ITEM	CALORIES	FAT	NET CARBS	PROTEIN

(Other Meals Eaten Today)

ITEM	CALORIES	FAT	NET CARBS	PROTEIN

[I Resumed Fasting At This Time]

Water Intake

What Went Well For Me Today

What Didn't Go Well For Me Today

How I Can Make It Better

FASTING & FOOD LOG

Date: ________________ [I Broke My Fast At: __________ a.m. p.m.]

M T W T F S S

Glucose-Ketone Index #

AM ....
MID-DAY ....
PM ....

["The earth is what we all have in common." Wendell Berry]

I Broke My Fast With...

ITEM	CALORIES	FAT	NET CARBS	PROTEIN

Other Meals Eaten Today

ITEM	CALORIES	FAT	NET CARBS	PROTEIN

Water Intake

I Resumed Fasting At This Time

What Went Well For Me Today

What Didn't Go Well For Me Today

How I Can Make It Better

FASTING & FOOD LOG

Date: ______________

M T W T F S S

[I Broke My Fast At: __________ a.m. p.m.]

Glucose-Ketone Index #

AM ....

MID-DAY ....

PM ....

["The wound is the place where the Light enters you." Rumi]

(I Broke My Fast With...)

ITEM	CALORIES	FAT	NET CARBS	PROTEIN

(Other Meals Eaten Today)

ITEM	CALORIES	FAT	NET CARBS	PROTEIN

[I Resumed Fasting At This Time]

Water Intake

What Went Well For Me Today

What Didn't Go Well For Me Today

How I Can Make It Better

FASTING & FOOD LOG

Glucose-Ketone Index #

AM ....

MID-DAY ....

PM ....

Date: ____________

[I Broke My Fast At: ________ a.m. p.m.]

M T W T F S S

["What happens when people open their hearts? They get better."]
Haruki Murakami

I Broke My Fast With...

ITEM	CALORIES	FAT	NET CARBS	PROTEIN

Other Meals Eaten Today

ITEM	CALORIES	FAT	NET CARBS	PROTEIN

Water Intake

[I Resumed Fasting At This Time]

What Went Well For Me Today

What Didn't Go Well For Me Today

How I Can Make It Better

FASTING & FOOD LOG

Glucose-Ketone Index #

AM ....

MID-DAY ....

PM ....

Date: ______________

[I Broke My Fast At: ________ a.m. p.m.]

M T W T F S S

["The emotion that can break your heart is sometimes the very one that heals it…"]
Nicholas Sparks

(I Broke My Fast With…)

ITEM	CALORIES	FAT	NET CARBS	PROTEIN

(Other Meals Eaten Today)

ITEM	CALORIES	FAT	NET CARBS	PROTEIN

Water Intake

[I Resumed Fasting At This Time]

What Went Well For Me Today

What Didn't Go Well For Me Today

How I Can Make It Better

FASTING & FOOD LOG

Date: ______________ [I Broke My Fast At: ________ a.m. p.m.]

M T W T F S S

Glucose-Ketone Index #

AM ....

MID-DAY ....

PM ....

["Our wounds are often the openings into the best and most beautiful part of us."]
David Richo

(I Broke My Fast With...)

ITEM	CALORIES	FAT	NET CARBS	PROTEIN

(Other Meals Eaten Today)

ITEM	CALORIES	FAT	NET CARBS	PROTEIN

Water Intake

[I Resumed Fasting At This Time]

What Went Well For Me Today

What Didn't Go Well For Me Today

How I Can Make It Better

FASTING & FOOD LOG

Glucose-Ketone Index #

AM ....

MID-DAY ....

PM ....

Date: ____________

[I Broke My Fast At: ________ a.m. p.m.]

M T W T F S S

["We are healed of a suffered only by experiencing it to the full." Marcel Proust]

I Broke My Fast With...

ITEM	CALORIES	FAT	NET CARBS	PROTEIN

Other Meals Eaten Today

ITEM	CALORIES	FAT	NET CARBS	PROTEIN

[I Resumed Fasting At This Time]

Water Intake

What Went Well For Me Today

What Didn't Go Well For Me Today

How I Can Make It Better

FASTING & FOOD LOG

Glucose-Ketone Index #

AM ....

MID-DAY ....

PM ....

Date: ______________

[I Broke My Fast At: ________ a.m. p.m.]

M T W T F S S

["Its when we start working together that the real healing takes place." David Hume]

(I Broke My Fast With...)

ITEM	CALORIES	FAT	NET CARBS	PROTEIN

(Other Meals Eaten Today)

ITEM	CALORIES	FAT	NET CARBS	PROTEIN

[I Resumed Fasting At This Time]

Water Intake

What Went Well For Me Today

What Didn't Go Well For Me Today

How I Can Make It Better

FASTING & FOOD LOG

Date: ______________

[I Broke My Fast At: ________ a.m. p.m.]

M T W T F S S

Glucose-Ketone Index #

AM ....

MID-DAY ....

PM ....

["Part of the healing process is sharing with other people who care." Jerry Cantrell]

(I Broke My Fast With...)

ITEM	CALORIES	FAT	NET CARBS	PROTEIN

(Other Meals Eaten Today)

ITEM	CALORIES	FAT	NET CARBS	PROTEIN

Water Intake

[I Resumed Fasting At This Time]

What Went Well For Me Today

What Didn't Go Well For Me Today

How I Can Make It Better

FASTING & FOOD LOG

Date: ______________

M T W T F S S

[I Broke My Fast At: ________ a.m. p.m.]

Glucose-Ketone Index #

AM ....

MID-DAY ....

PM ....

["The poison leaves bit by bit, not all at once. Be patient. You are healing."]
Yasmin Mogahed

(I Broke My Fast With...)

ITEM	CALORIES	FAT	NET CARBS	PROTEIN

(Other Meals Eaten Today)

ITEM	CALORIES	FAT	NET CARBS	PROTEIN

Water Intake

[I Resumed Fasting At This Time]

What Went Well For Me Today

What Didn't Go Well For Me Today

How I Can Make It Better

FASTING & FOOD LOG

Date: ______________

[I Broke My Fast At: ________ a.m. p.m.]

M T W T F S S

Glucose-Ketone Index #

AM ....

MID-DAY ....

PM ....

["You will will burn and you will burn out; you will be healed and come back again."]
Fyodor Dostoevsky

(I Broke My Fast With...)

ITEM	CALORIES	FAT	NET CARBS	PROTEIN

(Other Meals Eaten Today)

ITEM	CALORIES	FAT	NET CARBS	PROTEIN

Water Intake

[I Resumed Fasting At This Time]

What Went Well For Me Today

What Didn't Go Well For Me Today

How I Can Make It Better

FASTING & FOOD LOG

Date: ______________ [I Broke My Fast At: ________ a.m. p.m.]

M T W T F S S

Glucose-Ketone Index #

AM ....

MID-DAY ....

PM ....

["Healing in a matter of time, but it is sometimes also a matter of opportunity." Hippocrates]

(I Broke My Fast With...)

ITEM	CALORIES	FAT	NET CARBS	PROTEIN

(Other Meals Eaten Today)

ITEM	CALORIES	FAT	NET CARBS	PROTEIN

Water Intake

[I Resumed Fasting At This Time]

What Went Well For Me Today

What Didn't Go Well For Me Today

How I Can Make It Better

FASTING & FOOD LOG

Date: ________________

[I Broke My Fast At: __________ a.m. p.m.]

M T W T F S S

Glucose-Ketone Index #

AM ....

MID-DAY ....

PM ....

["You already have the precious mixture that will make you well. Use it." Rumi]

(I Broke My Fast With...)

ITEM	CALORIES	FAT	NET CARBS	PROTEIN

(Other Meals Eaten Today)

ITEM	CALORIES	FAT	NET CARBS	PROTEIN

[I Resumed Fasting At This Time]

Water Intake

What Went Well For Me Today

What Didn't Go Well For Me Today

How I Can Make It Better

FASTING & FOOD LOG

Date: ______________

[I Broke My Fast At: ________ a.m. p.m.]

M T W T F S S

Glucose-Ketone Index #	
AM	....
MID-DAY	....
PM	....

["Once you choose hope, anything's possible." Christopher Reeve]

(I Broke My Fast With...)

ITEM	CALORIES	FAT	NET CARBS	PROTEIN

(Other Meals Eaten Today)

ITEM	CALORIES	FAT	NET CARBS	PROTEIN

Water Intake

[I Resumed Fasting At This Time]

What Went Well For Me Today

What Didn't Go Well For Me Today

How I Can Make It Better

FASTING & FOOD LOG

Glucose-Ketone Index #

AM ....

MID-DAY ....

PM ....

Date: ______________

[I Broke My Fast At: ________ a.m. p.m.]

M T W T F S S

["Some people cannot be cured, but everyone can heal." Unknown]

I Broke My Fast With...

ITEM	CALORIES	FAT	NET CARBS	PROTEIN

Other Meals Eaten Today

ITEM	CALORIES	FAT	NET CARBS	PROTEIN

[I Resumed Fasting At This Time]

Water Intake

What Went Well For Me Today

What Didn't Go Well For Me Today

How I Can Make It Better

FASTING & FOOD LOG

Date: ______________

[I Broke My Fast At: __________ a.m. p.m.]

M T W T F S S

Glucose-Ketone Index #

AM ....

MID-DAY ....

PM ....

["Life isn't bout waiting for the storm to pass…It's about learning to dance in the rain."]
Vivian Greene

(I Broke My Fast With...)

ITEM	CALORIES	FAT	NET CARBS	PROTEIN

(Other Meals Eaten Today)

ITEM	CALORIES	FAT	NET CARBS	PROTEIN

Water Intake

[I Resumed Fasting At This Time]

What Went Well For Me Today

What Didn't Go Well For Me Today

How I Can Make It Better

FASTING & FOOD LOG

Glucose-Ketone Index #

AM ....

MID-DAY ....

PM ....

Date: ________________

[I Broke My Fast At: ________ a.m. p.m.]

M T W T F S S

["Love many, Trust few. Learn to paddle your own canoe." American Proverb]

(I Broke My Fast With...)

ITEM	CALORIES	FAT	NET CARBS	PROTEIN

(Other Meals Eaten Today)

ITEM	CALORIES	FAT	NET CARBS	PROTEIN

[I Resumed Fasting At This Time]

Water Intake

What Went Well For Me Today

What Didn't Go Well For Me Today

How I Can Make It Better

FASTING & FOOD LOG

Date: ______________

[I Broke My Fast At: ________ a.m. p.m.]

M T W T F S S

Glucose-Ketone Index #

AM ....

MID-DAY ....

PM ....

["The sun never quits shining. Sometimes, clouds just get in the way." Unknown]

(I Broke My Fast With...)

ITEM	CALORIES	FAT	NET CARBS	PROTEIN

(Other Meals Eaten Today)

ITEM	CALORIES	FAT	NET CARBS	PROTEIN

Water Intake

[I Resumed Fasting At This Time]

What Went Well For Me Today

What Didn't Go Well For Me Today

How I Can Make It Better

FASTING & FOOD LOG

Glucose-Ketone Index #

AM ....

MID-DAY ....

PM ....

Date: ________________

[I Broke My Fast At: ________ a.m. p.m.]

M T W T F S S

["Most folks are as happy as they make up their minds to be." Abraham Lincoln]

(I Broke My Fast With...)

ITEM	CALORIES	FAT	NET CARBS	PROTEIN

(Other Meals Eaten Today)

ITEM	CALORIES	FAT	NET CARBS	PROTEIN

[I Resumed Fasting At This Time]

Water Intake

What Went Well For Me Today

What Didn't Go Well For Me Today

How I Can Make It Better

FASTING & FOOD LOG

Glucose-Ketone Index #

AM ....

MID-DAY ....

PM ....

Date: ______________

[I Broke My Fast At: ________ a.m. p.m.]

M T W T F S S

["If there is life, there is hope." Stephen Hawking]

(I Broke My Fast With...)

ITEM	CALORIES	FAT	NET CARBS	PROTEIN

(Other Meals Eaten Today)

ITEM	CALORIES	FAT	NET CARBS	PROTEIN

[I Resumed Fasting At This Time]

Water Intake

What Went Well For Me Today

What Didn't Go Well For Me Today

How I Can Make It Better

FASTING & FOOD LOG

Date: ____________ [I Broke My Fast At: ________ a.m. p.m.]

M T W T F S S

Glucose-Ketone Index #

AM ....

MID-DAY ....

PM ....

["I don't know what the future may hold, but I know who holds the future." Ralph Abernathy]

(I Broke My Fast With...)

ITEM	CALORIES	FAT	NET CARBS	PROTEIN

(Other Meals Eaten Today)

ITEM	CALORIES	FAT	NET CARBS	PROTEIN

[I Resumed Fasting At This Time]

Water Intake

What Went Well For Me Today

What Didn't Go Well For Me Today

How I Can Make It Better

FASTING & FOOD LOG

Glucose-Ketone Index #	
AM	....
MID-DAY	....
PM	....

Date: ____________ [I Broke My Fast At: ________ a.m. p.m.]

M T W T F S S

["A smile doesn't cost a cent, but draws a lot of interest." Unknown]

(I Broke My Fast With...)

ITEM	CALORIES	FAT	NET CARBS	PROTEIN

(Other Meals Eaten Today)

ITEM	CALORIES	FAT	NET CARBS	PROTEIN

Water Intake

[I Resumed Fasting At This Time]

What Went Well For Me Today

What Didn't Go Well For Me Today

How I Can Make It Better

FASTING & FOOD LOG

Date: ______________

[I Broke My Fast At: __________ a.m. p.m.]

M T W T F S S

Glucose-Ketone Index #

AM ....

MID-DAY ....

PM ....

["The forces that are for you are greater than the forces against you." Joel Osteen]

(I Broke My Fast With...)

ITEM	CALORIES	FAT	NET CARBS	PROTEIN

(Other Meals Eaten Today)

ITEM	CALORIES	FAT	NET CARBS	PROTEIN

[I Resumed Fasting At This Time]

Water Intake

What Went Well For Me Today

What Didn't Go Well For Me Today

How I Can Make It Better

FASTING & FOOD LOG

Glucose-Ketone Index #

AM ....

MID-DAY ....

PM ....

Date: ______________

[I Broke My Fast At: ________ a.m. p.m.]

M T W T F S S

["And sometimes, against all odds, against all logic, we still hope." Ellen Pompeo]

(I Broke My Fast With...)

ITEM	CALORIES	FAT	NET CARBS	PROTEIN

(Other Meals Eaten Today)

ITEM	CALORIES	FAT	NET CARBS	PROTEIN

[I Resumed Fasting At This Time]

Water Intake

What Went Well For Me Today

What Didn't Go Well For Me Today

How I Can Make It Better

FASTING & FOOD LOG

Date: ____________ [I Broke My Fast At: ________ a.m. p.m.]

M T W T F S S

Glucose-Ketone Index #

AM ....

MID-DAY ....

PM ....

["Had to walk the rocks to see the mountain view." Caedmon's Call]

(I Broke My Fast With...)

ITEM	CALORIES	FAT	NET CARBS	PROTEIN

(Other Meals Eaten Today)

ITEM	CALORIES	FAT	NET CARBS	PROTEIN

Water Intake

[I Resumed Fasting At This Time]

What Went Well For Me Today

What Didn't Go Well For Me Today

How I Can Make It Better

FASTING & FOOD LOG

Glucose-Ketone Index #

AM ....
MID-DAY ....
PM ....

Date: ______________

[I Broke My Fast At: ________ a.m. p.m.]

M T W T F S S

["Let my love like sunlight surround you and yet give you illumined freedom."]
Rabindranath Tagore

(I Broke My Fast With...)

ITEM	CALORIES	FAT	NET CARBS	PROTEIN

(Other Meals Eaten Today)

ITEM	CALORIES	FAT	NET CARBS	PROTEIN

[I Resumed Fasting At This Time]

Water Intake

What Went Well For Me Today

What Didn't Go Well For Me Today

How I Can Make It Better

FASTING & FOOD LOG

Date: ______________

[I Broke My Fast At: ________ a.m. p.m.]

M T W T F S S

Glucose-Ketone Index #	
AM	....
MID-DAY	....
PM	....

["Being deeply loved by someone gives you strength, while loving someone deeply gives you courage."]
Lao Tzu

(I Broke My Fast With...)

ITEM	CALORIES	FAT	NET CARBS	PROTEIN

(Other Meals Eaten Today)

ITEM	CALORIES	FAT	NET CARBS	PROTEIN

Water Intake

[I Resumed Fasting At This Time]

What Went Well For Me Today

What Didn't Go Well For Me Today

How I Can Make It Better

FASTING & FOOD LOG

Date: ______________

[I Broke My Fast At: __________ a.m. p.m.]

M T W T F S S

Glucose-Ketone Index #

AM ....
MID-DAY ....
PM ....

["Healing takes courage, and we all have courage, even if we have to dig a little to find it."]
Tori Amos

(I Broke My Fast With...)

ITEM	CALORIES	FAT	NET CARBS	PROTEIN

(Other Meals Eaten Today)

ITEM	CALORIES	FAT	NET CARBS	PROTEIN

Water Intake

[I Resumed Fasting At This Time]

What Went Well For Me Today

What Didn't Go Well For Me Today

How I Can Make It Better

FASTING & FOOD LOG

Date: ______________

[I Broke My Fast At: __________ a.m. p.m.]

M T W T F S S

Glucose-Ketone Index #

AM ....

MID-DAY ....

PM ....

["The soul always knows what to do to heal itself. The challenge is to silence the mind."]
Caroline Myss

(I Broke My Fast With...)

ITEM	CALORIES	FAT	NET CARBS	PROTEIN

(Other Meals Eaten Today)

ITEM	CALORIES	FAT	NET CARBS	PROTEIN

Water Intake

[I Resumed Fasting At This Time]

What Went Well For Me Today

What Didn't Go Well For Me Today

How I Can Make It Better

FASTING & FOOD LOG

Date: ____________ [I Broke My Fast At: ________ a.m. p.m.]

M T W T F S S

Glucose-Ketone Index #

AM ....
MID-DAY ....
PM ....

["Self-forgiveness is essential to self-healing." Ruth Carter]

(I Broke My Fast With...)

ITEM	CALORIES	FAT	NET CARBS	PROTEIN

(Other Meals Eaten Today)

ITEM	CALORIES	FAT	NET CARBS	PROTEIN

Water Intake

[I Resumed Fasting At This Time]

What Went Well For Me Today

What Didn't Go Well For Me Today

How I Can Make It Better

FASTING & FOOD LOG

Glucose-Ketone Index #

AM ....

MID-DAY ....

PM ....

Date: ______________

[I Broke My Fast At: _________ a.m. p.m.]

M T W T F S S

["Healing yourself is connected with healing others." Yoko Ono]

(I Broke My Fast With...)

ITEM	CALORIES	FAT	NET CARBS	PROTEIN

(Other Meals Eaten Today)

ITEM	CALORIES	FAT	NET CARBS	PROTEIN

Water Intake

[I Resumed Fasting At This Time]

What Went Well For Me Today

What Didn't Go Well For Me Today

How I Can Make It Better

FASTING & FOOD LOG

Date: ______________

[I Broke My Fast At: __________ a.m. p.m.]

M T W T F S S

Glucose-Ketone Index #

AM ....

MID-DAY ....

PM ....

["Although the world is full of suffering, it is also full of the overcoming of it." Helen Keller]

(I Broke My Fast With...)

ITEM	CALORIES	FAT	NET CARBS	PROTEIN

(Other Meals Eaten Today)

ITEM	CALORIES	FAT	NET CARBS	PROTEIN

[I Resumed Fasting At This Time]

Water Intake

What Went Well For Me Today

What Didn't Go Well For Me Today

How I Can Make It Better

FASTING & FOOD LOG

Date: ______________

[I Broke My Fast At: __________ a.m. p.m.]

M T W T F S S

Glucose-Ketone Index #

AM ....

MID-DAY ....

PM ....

["Healing is an art. It takes time, it takes practice. It takes love." Maza Dohta]

(I Broke My Fast With...)

ITEM	CALORIES	FAT	NET CARBS	PROTEIN

(Other Meals Eaten Today)

ITEM	CALORIES	FAT	NET CARBS	PROTEIN

Water Intake

[I Resumed Fasting At This Time]

What Went Well For Me Today

What Didn't Go Well For Me Today

How I Can Make It Better

FASTING & FOOD LOG

Date: ____________ [I Broke My Fast At: ________ a.m. p.m.]

M T W T F S S

Glucose-Ketone Index #

AM ....

MID-DAY ....

PM ....

["When we heal the earth, we heal ourselves." David Orr]

I Broke My Fast With...

ITEM	CALORIES	FAT	NET CARBS	PROTEIN

Other Meals Eaten Today

ITEM	CALORIES	FAT	NET CARBS	PROTEIN

I Resumed Fasting At This Time

Water Intake

What Went Well For Me Today

What Didn't Go Well For Me Today

How I Can Make It Better

FASTING & FOOD LOG

Glucose-Ketone Index #

AM ....

MID-DAY ....

PM ....

Date: ______________

[I Broke My Fast At: ________ a.m. p.m.]

M T W T F S S

["Healing is an inside job." Dr. B.J. Palmer]

(I Broke My Fast With...)

ITEM	CALORIES	FAT	NET CARBS	PROTEIN

(Other Meals Eaten Today)

ITEM	CALORIES	FAT	NET CARBS	PROTEIN

Water Intake

[I Resumed Fasting At This Time]

What Went Well For Me Today

What Didn't Go Well For Me Today

How I Can Make It Better

FASTING & FOOD LOG

Date: ____________ [I Broke My Fast At: ________ a.m. p.m.]

M T W T F S S

Glucose-Ketone Index #

AM ....

MID-DAY ....

PM ....

["It's when we start working together that the real healing takes place." David Hume]

I Broke My Fast With...

ITEM	CALORIES	FAT	NET CARBS	PROTEIN

Other Meals Eaten Today

ITEM	CALORIES	FAT	NET CARBS	PROTEIN

Water Intake

[I Resumed Fasting At This Time]

What Went Well For Me Today

What Didn't Go Well For Me Today

How I Can Make It Better

FASTING & FOOD LOG

Date: ____________

[I Broke My Fast At: ________ a.m. p.m.]

M T W T F S S

Glucose-Ketone Index #

AM ....

MID-DAY ....

PM ....

["Natural forces within us are the true healers of disease." Hippocrates]

(I Broke My Fast With...)

ITEM	CALORIES	FAT	NET CARBS	PROTEIN

(Other Meals Eaten Today)

ITEM	CALORIES	FAT	NET CARBS	PROTEIN

[I Resumed Fasting At This Time]

Water Intake

What Went Well For Me Today

What Didn't Go Well For Me Today

How I Can Make It Better

FASTING & FOOD LOG

Date: ____________

M T W T F S S

[I Broke My Fast At: ________ a.m. p.m.]

Glucose-Ketone Index #

AM ....

MID-DAY ....

PM ....

["Every step taken in mindfulness brings us one step closer to healing ourselves and the planet."]
Thich Nhat Hanh

I Broke My Fast With...

ITEM	CALORIES	FAT	NET CARBS	PROTEIN

Other Meals Eaten Today

ITEM	CALORIES	FAT	NET CARBS	PROTEIN

Water Intake

[I Resumed Fasting At This Time]

What Went Well For Me Today

What Didn't Go Well For Me Today

How I Can Make It Better

FASTING & FOOD LOG

Date: ________ [I Broke My Fast At: ________ a.m. p.m.]

M T W T F S S

Glucose-Ketone Index #

AM ....

MID-DAY ....

PM ....

["Awareness is the first step in healing." Dean Ornish]

(I Broke My Fast With...)

ITEM	CALORIES	FAT	NET CARBS	PROTEIN

(Other Meals Eaten Today)

ITEM	CALORIES	FAT	NET CARBS	PROTEIN

[I Resumed Fasting At This Time]

Water Intake

What Went Well For Me Today

What Didn't Go Well For Me Today

How I Can Make It Better

FASTING & FOOD LOG

Date: ______________ [I Broke My Fast At: ________ a.m. p.m.]

M T W T F S S

Glucose-Ketone Index #

AM ....

MID-DAY ....

PM ....

["Of one thing I am certain, the body is not the measure of healing, peace is the measure."]
Phyllis McGinley

(I Broke My Fast With...)

ITEM	CALORIES	FAT	NET CARBS	PROTEIN

(Other Meals Eaten Today)

ITEM	CALORIES	FAT	NET CARBS	PROTEIN

Water Intake

[I Resumed Fasting At This Time]

What Went Well For Me Today

What Didn't Go Well For Me Today

How I Can Make It Better

FASTING & FOOD LOG

Glucose-Ketone Index #

AM ....

MID-DAY ....

PM ....

Date: ________________

[I Broke My Fast At: __________ a.m. p.m.]

M T W T F S S

["One of the healing things you can do is recognize where in your life you are your own poison." Steve Maraboli]

(I Broke My Fast With...)

ITEM	CALORIES	FAT	NET CARBS	PROTEIN

(Other Meals Eaten Today)

ITEM	CALORIES	FAT	NET CARBS	PROTEIN

[I Resumed Fasting At This Time]

Water Intake

What Went Well For Me Today

What Didn't Go Well For Me Today

How I Can Make It Better

FASTING & FOOD LOG

Date: ______________ [I Broke My Fast At: __________ a.m. p.m.]

M T W T F S S

Glucose-Ketone Index #

AM ....

MID-DAY ....

PM ....

["It's not all about healing yourself; it's just as importantly about letting yourself heal."]
Terri Guillemets

(I Broke My Fast With...)

ITEM	CALORIES	FAT	NET CARBS	PROTEIN

(Other Meals Eaten Today)

ITEM	CALORIES	FAT	NET CARBS	PROTEIN

Water Intake

[I Resumed Fasting At This Time]

What Went Well For Me Today

What Didn't Go Well For Me Today

How I Can Make It Better

FASTING & FOOD LOG

Date: ________________

[I Broke My Fast At: __________ a.m. p.m.]

M T W T F S S

Glucose-Ketone Index #

AM ....

MID-DAY ....

PM ....

["Ultimately, there can be no complete healing until we have restored our primal trust in life."]
George Feuerstein

(I Broke My Fast With...)

ITEM	CALORIES	FAT	NET CARBS	PROTEIN

(Other Meals Eaten Today)

ITEM	CALORIES	FAT	NET CARBS	PROTEIN

Water Intake

[I Resumed Fasting At This Time]

What Went Well For Me Today

What Didn't Go Well For Me Today

How I Can Make It Better

FASTING & FOOD LOG

Date: ______________ [I Broke My Fast At: ________ a.m. p.m.]

M T W T F S S

Glucose-Ketone Index #	
AM	....
MID-DAY	....
PM	....

["To heal is to touch with love that which we previously touched with fear." Stephen Levine]

(I Broke My Fast With...)

ITEM	CALORIES	FAT	NET CARBS	PROTEIN

(Other Meals Eaten Today)

ITEM	CALORIES	FAT	NET CARBS	PROTEIN

Water Intake

[I Resumed Fasting At This Time]

What Went Well For Me Today

What Didn't Go Well For Me Today

How I Can Make It Better

FASTING & FOOD LOG

Date: ____________

M T W T F S S

[I Broke My Fast At: ________ a.m. p.m.]

Glucose-Ketone Index #

AM ....

MID-DAY ....

PM ....

["Progress and healing involves seeing every person as not so different from ourselves."]
Bryant H. McGill

(I Broke My Fast With...)

ITEM	CALORIES	FAT	NET CARBS	PROTEIN

(Other Meals Eaten Today)

ITEM	CALORIES	FAT	NET CARBS	PROTEIN

Water Intake

[I Resumed Fasting At This Time]

What Went Well For Me Today

What Didn't Go Well For Me Today

How I Can Make It Better

FASTING & FOOD LOG

Glucose-Ketone Index #

AM ....

MID-DAY ....

PM ....

Date: ______________

[I Broke My Fast At: __________ a.m. p.m.]

M T W T F S S

["Out of suffering have emerged the strongest souls; the most massive characters are seared with scars."
Kahlil Gibran]

(I Broke My Fast With...)

ITEM	CALORIES	FAT	NET CARBS	PROTEIN

(Other Meals Eaten Today)

ITEM	CALORIES	FAT	NET CARBS	PROTEIN

[I Resumed Fasting At This Time]

Water Intake

What Went Well For Me Today

What Didn't Go Well For Me Today

How I Can Make It Better

FASTING & FOOD LOG

Date: ____________ [I Broke My Fast At: ________ a.m. p.m.]

M T W T F S S

Glucose-Ketone Index #

AM ....

MID-DAY ....

PM ....

["We do not heal the past by dwelling there; we heal the past by living in the present."]
Marianne Williamson

(I Broke My Fast With...)

ITEM	CALORIES	FAT	NET CARBS	PROTEIN

(Other Meals Eaten Today)

ITEM	CALORIES	FAT	NET CARBS	PROTEIN

Water Intake

[I Resumed Fasting At This Time]

What Went Well For Me Today

What Didn't Go Well For Me Today

How I Can Make It Better

FASTING & FOOD LOG

Date: ______________ [I Broke My Fast At: _________ a.m. p.m.]

M T W T F S S

Glucose-Ketone Index #

AM ....

MID-DAY ....

PM ....

["There are two ways of spreading light: to be the candle or the mirror that reflects it."]
Edith Wharton

I Broke My Fast With...

ITEM	CALORIES	FAT	NET CARBS	PROTEIN

Other Meals Eaten Today

ITEM	CALORIES	FAT	NET CARBS	PROTEIN

Water Intake

[I Resumed Fasting At This Time]

What Went Well For Me Today

What Didn't Go Well For Me Today

How I Can Make It Better

FASTING & FOOD LOG

Glucose-Ketone Index #

AM ....

MID-DAY ....

PM ....

Date: ____________________

[I Broke My Fast At: __________ a.m. p.m.]

M T W T F S S

["You do not find the happy life. You make it." Camilla Eyring Kimbal]

(I Broke My Fast With...)

ITEM	CALORIES	FAT	NET CARBS	PROTEIN

(Other Meals Eaten Today)

ITEM	CALORIES	FAT	NET CARBS	PROTEIN

[I Resumed Fasting At This Time]

Water Intake

What Went Well For Me Today

What Didn't Go Well For Me Today

How I Can Make It Better

FASTING & FOOD LOG

Glucose-Ketone Index #

AM ....

MID-DAY ....

PM ....

Date: ______________

[I Broke My Fast At: ________ a.m. p.m.]

M T W T F S S

["The most wasted of days is one without laughter." E. E. Cummings]

(I Broke My Fast With...)

ITEM	CALORIES	FAT	NET CARBS	PROTEIN

(Other Meals Eaten Today)

ITEM	CALORIES	FAT	NET CARBS	PROTEIN

[I Resumed Fasting At This Time]

Water Intake

What Went Well For Me Today

What Didn't Go Well For Me Today

How I Can Make It Better

FASTING & FOOD LOG

Date: ______________ [I Broke My Fast At: ________ a.m. p.m.]

M T W T F S S

Glucose-Ketone Index #

AM ....

MID-DAY ....

PM ....

["Stay close to anything that makes you glad you are alive." Hafez]

I Broke My Fast With...

ITEM	CALORIES	FAT	NET CARBS	PROTEIN

Other Meals Eaten Today

ITEM	CALORIES	FAT	NET CARBS	PROTEIN

Water Intake

[I Resumed Fasting At This Time]

What Went Well For Me Today

What Didn't Go Well For Me Today

How I Can Make It Better

FASTING & FOOD LOG

Date: ____________

[I Broke My Fast At: ________ a.m. p.m.]

M T W T F S S

Glucose-Ketone Index #

AM ....

MID-DAY ....

PM ....

["Make each day your masterpiece." John Wooden]

(I Broke My Fast With...)

ITEM	CALORIES	FAT	NET CARBS	PROTEIN

(Other Meals Eaten Today)

ITEM	CALORIES	FAT	NET CARBS	PROTEIN

Water Intake

[I Resumed Fasting At This Time]

What Went Well For Me Today

What Didn't Go Well For Me Today

How I Can Make It Better

FASTING & FOOD LOG

Glucose-Ketone Index #

AM ....

MID-DAY ....

PM ....

Date: ________________

[I Broke My Fast At: __________ a.m. p.m.]

M T W T F S S

["Happiness often sneaks in through a door you didn't know you left open." John Barrymore]

(I Broke My Fast With...)

ITEM	CALORIES	FAT	NET CARBS	PROTEIN

(Other Meals Eaten Today)

ITEM	CALORIES	FAT	NET CARBS	PROTEIN

[I Resumed Fasting At This Time]

Water Intake

What Went Well For Me Today

What Didn't Go Well For Me Today

How I Can Make It Better

FASTING & FOOD LOG

Date: ______________ [I Broke My Fast At: ________ a.m. p.m.]

M T W T F S S

Glucose-Ketone Index #

AM ....

MID-DAY ....

PM ....

["Happiness is not by chance, but by choice." Jim Rohn]

(I Broke My Fast With...)

ITEM	CALORIES	FAT	NET CARBS	PROTEIN

(Other Meals Eaten Today)

ITEM	CALORIES	FAT	NET CARBS	PROTEIN

Water Intake

[I Resumed Fasting At This Time]

What Went Well For Me Today

What Didn't Go Well For Me Today

How I Can Make It Better

FASTING & FOOD LOG

Date: ____________

M T W T F S S

[I Broke My Fast At: ________ a.m. p.m.]

Glucose-Ketone Index #	
AM	....
MID-DAY	....
PM	....

["Life changes quickly, in a very positive way, if you let it." Lindsey Vonn]

(I Broke My Fast With...)

ITEM	CALORIES	FAT	NET CARBS	PROTEIN

(Other Meals Eaten Today)

ITEM	CALORIES	FAT	NET CARBS	PROTEIN

Water Intake

[I Resumed Fasting At This Time]

What Went Well For Me Today

What Didn't Go Well For Me Today

How I Can Make It Better

FASTING & FOOD LOG

Date: ______________

M T W T F S S

[I Broke My Fast At: ________ a.m. p.m.]

Glucose-Ketone Index #

AM ....

MID-DAY ....

PM ....

["Impossible is for the unwilling." John Keats]

(I Broke My Fast With...)

ITEM	CALORIES	FAT	NET CARBS	PROTEIN

(Other Meals Eaten Today)

ITEM	CALORIES	FAT	NET CARBS	PROTEIN

Water Intake

[I Resumed Fasting At This Time]

What Went Well For Me Today

What Didn't Go Well For Me Today

How I Can Make It Better

FASTING & FOOD LOG

Date: ______________

[I Broke My Fast At: ________ a.m. p.m.]

M T W T F S S

Glucose-Ketone Index #

AM ....

MID-DAY ....

PM ....

["Believe you can and you're halfway there." Theodore Roosevelt]

(I Broke My Fast With...)

ITEM	CALORIES	FAT	NET CARBS	PROTEIN

(Other Meals Eaten Today)

ITEM	CALORIES	FAT	NET CARBS	PROTEIN

Water Intake

[I Resumed Fasting At This Time]

What Went Well For Me Today

What Didn't Go Well For Me Today

How I Can Make It Better

FASTING & FOOD LOG

Glucose-Ketone Index #

AM ....

MID-DAY ....

PM ....

Date: ______________

[I Broke My Fast At: ________ a.m. p.m.]

M T W T F S S

["Failure is the condiment that gives success its flavor." Truman Capote]

I Broke My Fast With...

ITEM	CALORIES	FAT	NET CARBS	PROTEIN

Other Meals Eaten Today

ITEM	CALORIES	FAT	NET CARBS	PROTEIN

Water Intake

[I Resumed Fasting At This Time]

What Went Well For Me Today

What Didn't Go Well For Me Today

How I Can Make It Better

FASTING & FOOD LOG

Date: ____________ [I Broke My Fast At: ________ a.m. p.m.]

M T W T F S S

Glucose-Ketone Index #

AM ....

MID-DAY ....

PM ....

["It is never too late to be what you might have been." George Eliot]

(I Broke My Fast With...)

ITEM	CALORIES	FAT	NET CARBS	PROTEIN

(Other Meals Eaten Today)

ITEM	CALORIES	FAT	NET CARBS	PROTEIN

Water Intake

[I Resumed Fasting At This Time]

What Went Well For Me Today

What Didn't Go Well For Me Today

How I Can Make It Better

FASTING & FOOD LOG

Glucose-Ketone Index #

AM ....

MID-DAY ....

PM ....

Date: ______________

[I Broke My Fast At: __________ a.m. p.m.]

M T W T F S S

["You must do the things you think you cannot do." Eleanor Roosevelt]

(I Broke My Fast With...)

ITEM	CALORIES	FAT	NET CARBS	PROTEIN

(Other Meals Eaten Today)

ITEM	CALORIES	FAT	NET CARBS	PROTEIN

[I Resumed Fasting At This Time]

Water Intake

What Went Well For Me Today

What Didn't Go Well For Me Today

How I Can Make It Better

FASTING & FOOD LOG

Date: ______________

[I Broke My Fast At: __________ a.m. p.m.]

M T W T F S S

Glucose-Ketone Index #

AM ....

MID-DAY ....

PM ....

["Be faithful to that which exists within yourself." Andre Gide]

(I Broke My Fast With...)

ITEM	CALORIES	FAT	NET CARBS	PROTEIN

(Other Meals Eaten Today)

ITEM	CALORIES	FAT	NET CARBS	PROTEIN

Water Intake

[I Resumed Fasting At This Time]

What Went Well For Me Today

What Didn't Go Well For Me Today

How I Can Make It Better

FASTING & FOOD LOG

Glucose-Ketone Index #

AM ....

MID-DAY ....

PM ....

Date: ______________

[I Broke My Fast At: ________ a.m. p.m.]

M T W T F S S

["My mission in life is not merely to survive, but to thrive." Maya Angelou]

(I Broke My Fast With...)

ITEM	CALORIES	FAT	NET CARBS	PROTEIN

(Other Meals Eaten Today)

ITEM	CALORIES	FAT	NET CARBS	PROTEIN

[I Resumed Fasting At This Time]

Water Intake

What Went Well For Me Today

What Didn't Go Well For Me Today

How I Can Make It Better

FASTING & FOOD LOG

Glucose-Ketone Index #

AM ....

MID-DAY ....

PM ....

Date: ______________

[I Broke My Fast At: ________ a.m. p.m.]

M T W T F S S

["To be the best, you must be able to handle the worst." Wilson Kanadi]

(I Broke My Fast With...)

ITEM	CALORIES	FAT	NET CARBS	PROTEIN

(Other Meals Eaten Today)

ITEM	CALORIES	FAT	NET CARBS	PROTEIN

[I Resumed Fasting At This Time]

Water Intake

What Went Well For Me Today

What Didn't Go Well For Me Today

How I Can Make It Better

FASTING & FOOD LOG

Date: ______________ [I Broke My Fast At: __________ a.m. p.m.]

M T W T F S S

Glucose-Ketone Index #

AM ....

MID-DAY ....

PM ....

["Nothing is impossible. The word itself says "I'm possible!"." Audrey Hepburn]

(I Broke My Fast With...)

ITEM	CALORIES	FAT	NET CARBS	PROTEIN

(Other Meals Eaten Today)

ITEM	CALORIES	FAT	NET CARBS	PROTEIN

Water Intake

[I Resumed Fasting At This Time]

What Went Well For Me Today

What Didn't Go Well For Me Today

How I Can Make It Better

FASTING & FOOD LOG

Glucose-Ketone Index #

AM ....

MID-DAY ....

PM ....

Date: ________________

[I Broke My Fast At: __________ a.m. p.m.]

M T W T F S S

[Don't Give Up. You Can Do This]

(I Broke My Fast With...)

ITEM	CALORIES	FAT	NET CARBS	PROTEIN

(Other Meals Eaten Today)

ITEM	CALORIES	FAT	NET CARBS	PROTEIN

Water Intake

[I Resumed Fasting At This Time]

What Went Well For Me Today

What Didn't Go Well For Me Today

How I Can Make It Better

Made in the USA
Monee, IL
08 November 2026

67971103R00109